Using cosmetics? I bet you don't know how!

A user manual for the regular man – your skin has one too

by

Davor Pavlić

2018

Table of Contents

INTRODUCTION

Welcome to the Cosmetics handbook.

This handbook is a set of advice, written while researching the benefits and downsides of certain ingredients for hair and skin.

Some of the information may only be men specific, but there is information here that can be used by everyone and it would be beneficial for everyone to read. It will come as a surprise to you that many of us don't even wash or dry our hair properly and then complain about the damage it has endured.

Most, but not all of this information, is available on the internet if you have time or patience to do a thorough research. But given that internet is filled with a lot of junk also, I would advise against it and suggest you invest in knowing how to take care of yourself. Not only with this handbook, but in general.

History of cosmetics

If we were to compare it to its origins, cosmetics products as we know them do not exist for a very long time and in the last 100 or so years they were changing faster than in history because the styles were also changing each decade.

But where did it all start? Well, I couldn't really give you a definitive answer. It seems that even in the Copper age paint has been used for making tattoos. But for the purposes of smelling nice and looking better it has been used since ancient Egypt. Once the cosmetics started spreading outside of Egypt it wasn't as widely accepted. Just like today, there were people and societies who thought that it was not needed and extravagant. But eventually it got accepted and women were even considered not beautiful if they didn't have any cosmetics. A Roman philosopher Plautus once said that "A woman without paint is like food without salt".

From those advanced ancient cultures all the way to the dark ages all civilizations knew some sort of cosmetics, be it as a sign of wealth and nobility or Spartan soldiers getting ready for battle. Many of them actually promoted cleanliness. Until kings and Church started rumors that cosmetics were used by Satan worshipers and for the most time it was reserved for actors. The lack of the use of cosmetics went so far into the negative that it even became popular to have bad hygiene. For example, it was popular to have bad teeth and the reason for this was that bad teeth were tied to wealth because only wealthy people could pay for sugar. It went so far that some people even used ash to fake bad teeth.

So, it started with jewelry and oils, then it went on to lead being used to keep an appearance of pale complexion, sometimes women didn't even go out into the direct sunlight to avoid getting darker, since that would mean they were working in the fields… How the times have changed. Tans became popular in 1920's and the sun tan bed was invented in 1978.

Now, I do not want to go in too much depth about the history of cosmetics even though the title says exactly that. The point of this article is to get a message across to everyone who may oppose cosmetics. It is not a novelty thing and it is not used for centuries, it is used for millennia. Even the absence of cosmetics when people were darkening their teeth to look like they weren't healthy was actually cosmetics.

Having bad teeth, hair or skin just because you are scared you will not be manly enough is not worth it. There is nothing masculine about bad skin, bald patch on your head or any other condition that could actually be prevented. While we could argue that some men take it a bit too far, this is no reason for you to go to the absolute opposite extreme to prove to someone that you are not like that. You have nothing to prove to anyone, but yourself. I really suggest you keep reading this and especially the article about what products men should be using if you are still conflicted.

What cosmetic products should men be using

Since we all have different conditions through different races and different age groups and live in different parts of the world with different weather, it would be very presumptuous of me to claim that I have some ultimate solution and a certain number of products that one just MUST use. Well, I don't and anyone who says they do, they are lying.

However, there are some directions that we may tackle and try to get to a solution of this problem or at least give you enough guidelines so you can solve it for yourself.

Hopefully you are shaving. You may like your beard and I won't judge you for your choice, it is my personal preference not to have one. One reason is that it's more hygienic and the other is that I don't want my skin to become even more sensitive than it already is. I have had some breaks from not shaving and then when I got back to it, the rash that followed was horrible.

So what would you need for a proper shave? And I do mean proper, not something you do in two minutes. This would be what I am using: a shaving cream (not gel, not foam, not soap) combined with a pre-shave cream or oil; a double edge safety razor or if you're feeling brave a straight razor; a shaving brush; a face wash; some kind of after shave, I think I prefer balm over the alcohol rich liquid ones; and the styptic pencil.

Let me explain this.
You want your face and your beard to soften up, so you wash it in warm water with a face wash, maybe even a scrub. You want your face clean of any bacteria, since cuts happen. If you happen to cut yourself, don't reach for toilet paper to stick it to your face, that is what

the styptic is for. Put it under a tap and then go over the cut. It stings, but it works. I also recommend using the shaving cream and brush. Cream because those usually don't come in pressurized containers and are better for the environment and your skin and the brush because it can lift up your beard for cutting it, instead of flattening it with your palm while putting on the gel. I use the pre-shave products just for added benefit, but it's not a must. The double edge safety razor or the straight razor are better because they only have one edge. You do not want to shave too many times over a surface that has no shaving cream on it. So, the fewer blades, the better. Personally, I put the shaving cream on three times before I am done. First time it's the regular top to bottom shave. Second time it's side to side shave. And the third time it's bottom up shave. After this process, you can wash your face and inspect for any cuts and if you missed any spots that need fixing and then you apply your choice of after shave.

Bonus product: if you let the beard grow too much out, you may want to use a trimmer of some kind to make it shorter, so you have an easier shave.

Regular face routine, without shaving, should also be mentioned because too often we as men neglect it and use whatever is handy. A bar of soap that we use for everything else? Just think about what that soap has touched… I hope not. And that can often be the end of our care for our face. Now, I'm not suggest you start using face masks, even though I don't have anything against those, but something more should be done. You should have at least three products: a face wash (can be the same as the one you use for preparation for shaving); a face scrub; face cream. I'll elaborate on the cream a bit more next.

I'm not sure if there is anything special to say here. Explaining how to wash your face? That must sound ridiculous. Let's see… I never advise using the face wash on a dry face. First a splash of water, then a smaller amount of face wash, rubbing it in gently, leave for a few seconds if you want and then wash it out. There are brushes some use for washing your face, even automated tools, but I don't use any of those. After this, if you are using a cream with an SPF factor, which would make it a day cream, you do not want your face to be gun powder dry. You put on the cream on a mildly wet face. Most of the creams have ingredients that keep moisture, so give them something to lock in. Also, the creams spread better when the face isn't completely dry, so you actually save on the cream and can save some money there. If you are using a scrub, and I suggest you do, you don't need to use it daily, it would be enough to use it 2-3 times a week.

Bonus: Tweezers. Even though this part is about cleaning, you don't want to have a monobrow or some rogue hairs, so pluck them out. And eyebrows you want to pluck and not shave or it will just grow out much worse with a thicker end.

Bonus 2: Lip balm. If you're avoiding it just because it's not masculine enough, don't worry. They are made in some masculine packaging also, some are much bigger than the rest or come in flavours like whiskey. It wouldn't make sense for you to take good care of your face and forget about the lips. They are on your face, you know. And if you're planning to have a second kiss after the first one, I suggest you take better care of that sandpaper on your face.

Let's talk about hair products next. Similar to our care about our face, we don't care about our hair either until it's very late or even too late. What do we use? Cheap shampoos, cheap styling products and probably nothing more. Most men probably never turned the bottle to see what they are actually putting on their heads. So, what are the products we should be using for our hair? Let's see… Shampoo, conditioner, styling products. I hope I don't need to say anything about hair dryers or combs here.

So, in total there is actually quite a number of products on this list that every man should use. And that's not taking into account things like toothpaste etc. While I can give you guidelines what you should do, you still need to do your own research of what products suit you best and if you need more. Maybe apart from the products I mentioned you also could use an eye cream or something extra for the acne or something else. That is the individual part that you will need to find out for yourself or discuss it with your dermatologist.

HAIR

How to prevent hair loss

Hair loss is something that many men will face at some point in their lives. Male pattern baldness can start as early as 21 years old or younger. Two thirds of men will experience some hair loss by the age of 35. Over 800.000 people each year seek some sort of treatment for the hair loss. Two more statistics are very interesting. The decade you are in equals the chance of the hair loss – e.g. if you are in your 20's you have 20% chance for hair loss, etc. The other one is that 50% of the hair is gone before we even start noticing it. And one I will give you for free… 100% men never said I'm glad I started losing hair.

Some drugs for certain conditions can cause hair loss, but you don't really want to stop using those until you are feeling better. Too much styling of your hair can cause hair loss. Hair treatment is becoming more popular with men too, so bleaching, chemical treatments and heated tools can cause falling out. So, are there ways to prevent hair loss? Yes and no. We can fight some of it, but some of it is just genetical and is caused by us being men – hormones, or testosterone to be specific. Speaking of drugs, there are some treatments that would supposedly help with your hair, but some of those drugs have nasty side-effects. Post-finasteride syndrome is a condition brought on by a drug named 5-alpha reductase type II. The drug is meant to stop hair loss and prevent the body from rejecting transplanted hair. The drug is halting something else too. Namely, erection in men. It is also tied to muscle atrophy, fatigue, depression (who wouldn't be), reduction of semen and some other conditions. Another popular treatment is Rogaine and there is a cheaper brand on the market also, I think it's Kirkland. The active ingredient here is Minoxidil and while the foam can be quite effective faster than most other treatments, when you stop using it its effects subside faster as well. It also can cause redness etc. A slower ingredient is Stemoxidine, but its effects last longer and aren't as aggressive.

Before I start with listing anything about how to prevent or slow down the thinning of your hair, I want to point out that once you start noticing this, you may want to do a regular check-up with your doctor. It may not be anything, but… Hair loss can be the visible manifestation of some other health issues you may or may not have. With men it could be linked to the prostate or coronary issues. Hair loss could even be the cause of some health issues, such as depression and anxiety. But, even if everything is OK with you, a regular check-up is always good and a chance to consult with your doctor if there is anything that you should or shouldn't use and not self medicate.

Some things I point out may not seem like a lot to you, but combine them into one and the impact or the difference may be noticeable. So, let's start with this.

Learn how to wash your hair. We men don't really think much about washing our hair. Get into the shower, turn water on, get wet, put shampoo on, wash out, dry, comb, done. Well, it's not that simple. You can read the article about how to wash your hair later, so we don't make this one too long.

Have you noticed more hair falling out after using a certain styling product? Maybe it's not the end of the world. Our hair falls out daily. And when we use any product really, it can possibly damage our hair. Rarely will they cause the falling out of our hair. But what can happen is if you kept the product in your hair for a day or maybe even two, the hair that has fallen out before, it may stick to the hair that hasn't. So once you wash your hair after the break you get the effect of hair falling out more because it's maybe a two-three days worth.

I'm not saying you do not have a problem. You may have. Many men will have this at some point in their lives. But this is something to take into consideration. There are also some products you may use to prevent the hair falling out.

Just using better tools to comb your hair will be helpful as well. This may be a ludacris thing to spend the money on, but I would say no matter how much money you spend on a comb or looking for one that suits you, it will still be less than many expensive procedures to try and get your hair back. You could use a wooden wide tooth comb after washing your hair. The reason for this is because your hair may be tangled up from washing. Especially if your hair is a bit longer. After you have untangled your hair you can use something finer, it's just important to prevent the tugging. ***Do not go to bed with wet hair.*** Pulling on the hair that didn't dry could actually help lose a bit more hair than you would, the hair is the weakest when it is wet.

I won't talk much about **food** in this article, as I have another one only about what food is good for you, but let's just say that some multivitamins and minerals are also used as a treatment for hair loss. The best known one in the States seems to be HR23+.

Some even use derma rollers on their head. These are devices with small needles used usually on the face to promote collagen production, but some have found it effective for promoting hair growth as well.

You cannot do only one thing and expect an overnight change. You can not work only from the outside using a decent shampoo and not work from the inside – using foods, drinks, exercising, meditating, sleeping well… If we just take these examples, you are doing only 1/6th of the work by using a good shampoo. Yes, I'm sure it will help, but you could do so much more.

Dandruff

What is dandruff? It is a condition that is marked by flaking of the skin on your scalp and is sometimes accompanied by itchiness. Dandruff isn't contagious and you can't get it from someone else, other than on your clothes if you lend a jacket to a person who has it. It certainly can be a bit embarrassing, especially if you go out somewhere where they have UV lights. I certainly hope that dandruff will be the only thing that will glow.

There are several risk factors when talking about dandruff. *Age* is one of those factors. Usually dandruff appears at young age and can continue through some later periods in life, which is also another reason to use quality products for your hair. *Sex* seems to be an issue to, since dandruff appears more with men. Flakes from *dry skin* are generally smaller and less oily than those from other causes of dandruff. And, redness or inflammation is unlikely. You'll probably have dry skin on other parts of the body, such as your legs and arms, too. *Oily hair and scalp* is another issue. Malassezia feeds on oils in your scalp. For that reason, having excessively oily skin and hair makes you more prone to dandruff. For reasons that aren't clear, adults with neurological *diseases*, such as Parkinson's disease, are more likely to develop seborrheic dermatitis and dandruff. So are people with HIV infection, or those who have compromised immune systems from other conditions. Sometimes *sensitivity to certain ingredients* in hair care products or hair dyes can cause a red, itchy, scaly scalp.

The good thing about dandruff is that most cases aren't that extreme. Mild cases may be solved with only daily shampooing. Some of the more stubborn ones may need some prescribed shampoos.

I will go out on a limb here and say that you shouldn't use any natural treatments for dandruff. Especially when you read that a website I don't even want to name to generate even one more visitors lists the following as natural treatment: aspirin, mouth wash, baking soda… Really?! Even if you consider how we make oils, you could argue how natural those are. Please, leave the food off your hair and eat it, work from the inside as well and find a good shampoo that will treat your problem. Other than that, tone down the use of any extra products you may be putting in your hair.

Research into ways to help people with psoriasis and other skin conditions is ongoing. Green tea has shown potential for the treatment of dandruff and psoriasis, according to research published in 2012. Researchers believe a special formulation that can penetrate the skin's waterproof barrier will combat excessive cell growth, oxidative stress, and inflammation. A study carried out by European researchers has suggested that the addition of llama antibodies to shampoo could be a new strategy for fighting dandruff.

How to wash your hair

What do you need to know about washing your hair? A lot. Men usually think it's as simple as going into the shower, turn water on, get wet, put shampoo on, rinse, dry, comb, done. It's a bit more complicated and this process starts way before you get into the shower.

First of all, you need to find a product that is good for your hair, so a quality shampoo. You may not want to spend money on it now, but once you start losing hair you'll be sorry you haven't and it will be cheap in comparison to the treatment for hair loss. Many of the shampoos will claim that they help hair growth or prevent hair loss, but then they contain ingredients like parabens. Parabens will basically prevent or at least limit the benefit that the shampoo would have done to your hair if there weren't any in it.

Men will often only buy a shampoo. We don't even have a word 'conditioner' in our vocabulary for a very long time, I don't think. But this is the second product you will buy and use. If possible, my advice would be to have them from the same company if they are quality products. But in the process of finding something that suits you, you may find different products and combine them.

Now you can finally step into the shower.

Water… The temperature shouldn't be too hot. Same as using heated tools or blow drying into the scalp it can be damaging to the scalp and hair, so the water should be somewhere in the middle. If you can take a few seconds of cold water at the end, that is not bad either. Just go slowly, don't go from hot to totally cold in one second. This will help your circulation a little bit too.

Rubbing the shampoo in… I have seen people rub the shampoo with their whole palm, pulling and tugging the hair. The correct way of doing this would be with your fingertips pushing down and up. Also, this should be done as gently as possible, your hair will not be any cleaner if your grip is harder.

How many times should you shampoo your hair… One or two, not more. Personally, until I get my own shampoo I use two different ones, so this isn't even an option. When mine is done I may still stick with two times, but if you feel once is enough, then that is OK. Remember that the last one will always be your conditioner. I can not explain in short what it does for your hair, but trust me, it's good. Untangling, nurturing, protecting, returning what detergents from shampoo stripped… it does help. But still, don't be too generous with the shampoo. Over shampooing won't cause you to lose hair, but it could cause some other issues that you would rather avoid.

You will not believe this, but ***there is even order in which you should use the product***. OK, we all know that conditioner comes after the shampoo. I hope. But even I only recently found out that it is advised to wash your body after you wash your hair. This is because you will be washing the shampoo off your body more thoroughly and you will be removing any harmful ingredients that may cause you to have some reaction to it. And this is why you should avoid using products that claim to be both, a shampoo and a body wash. There is no such things, our scalp and our body have different pH values.

Drying your hair… Same as rubbing the shampoo in. You should not be drying your hair with a towel like you want to pull it out of your head. The correct way to towel dry your hair would be to place the towel over your head and gently move it through the hair. Imagine you came across a child and you ruffle through his hair. This is what you will be doing to yourself, but over a towel. You shouldn't really feel any pressure on your scalp.

Now we come to styling your hair… Wait a second, put something on first!!! First you would comb your hair with a wide tooth wooden comb. This is used to untangle your hair in case it gets tangled for those of you with a bit longer hair. After that you can use a finer brush or a tool of your choice, maybe a finer tooth comb and then style it to your liking.

Few points about styling… I left out blow drying your hair in the paragraph above because it is often used together with styling. When blow drying your hair you should never feel the heat on your scalp. Basically, *the hot air should be flowing over your head and not into it.* But in any case, I don't do it every time I style my hair and I would also recommend that you skip it from time to time. It can add volume if you need it, though.

Depending on the length of your hair you may have issues controlling it. I do hope you don't and if you do, maybe you can use something to constrain it, hold it in place. I do not like to put any product in my hair right after washing it because I like to give the hair also a period to rest and not always have something in it. I will do it only if I'm going out or if styling it just with blow drying really doesn't work.

The products you are using should be water soluble. This will help you to wash out the product without using heavy shampoos. And this will help you with your hair washing schedule. Well, maybe not a schedule, but you shouldn't really be washing it more than 3 times a week. Hair needs rest, even from shampoos and water, not just styling products.

Correct way of styling your hair

Let's first cover what the hair should be like... *Most of the time it's good to work with wet or damp hair. I rarely work with dry hair.* I will however work with dry hair if I want that true matt finish right away and I am in a hurry, so I can not blow dry my hair and if I have some paste that is relatively easy to spread through dry hair. Other than that the procedure would be as follows.

Like I said, I do not recommend styling your hair right after you have washed it. So, when styling *just wet the palms of your hands with water and run them through your hair.* It will make it damp enough. Additionally, if you have a prestyler with some sort of heat protection I usually don't spray it on the hair, I spray it into my palm and spread it just like I did with water or any product.

After your hair is damp enough before any kind of products you should *finger comb first.* Even if you will mess it up a little bit later it's good to have some of the hairstyle done before you apply the product. This is important because it will untangle your hair for combing and because some of the products have a higher hold and the effect steps in very fast, that's the case with clays usually.

Blow drying your hair and combing it after you are done with styling is not something I do every time, but it is good to do if you want to add a little bit of volume to your hair. But if you do not have these issues I would recommend you skip blow drying once in a while at least.

For some extra hold you could eventually use some liquid gel or something, but the less products you use on your hair, the better. If you can't find a good liquid gel, but have the normal version of it, you could turn it into liquid by adding table salt to it. Not sure how much this would be advised, but since some pre-stylers are actually sea salt, I guess you can go ahead and do it.

Hair styling tools

We as men usually don't need too many tools to get our hair done, but we can make ourselves familiar with a few different ones and what each of those will help us achieve.

As men we don't really take too much interest in various tools unless we're hairdressers or really enthusiastic about our hair, but I can tell you one thing – there's more than just a comb. So, by now you have more than likely heard about *combs*. They are very widespread, they are usually very cheap and they can differ in the width of the space between the teeth and the material they are made of. Comb is also one of the wider tools that have been used in making ourselves look better and it is purely manual. On the other hand, there are also *brushes*, which can be manual and automated. Another very crude difference is that there are paddle brushes and round brushes. Round or semi-round are used to make shapes and curls.

If you're using a fine boar hair bristle brush you'll be glad to find out that it also removes dust, flakes and hair product from your hair. Not only does it clean, it can even help you spread the natural oils across your hair.

And while the brush is usually used on dry hair for cleaning and spreading of the natural oils, combs are more often used on wet or damp hair for untangling the hair and for styling. This is usually the problem that women face, but some men have long hair too… You may want to gradually narrow the width of the comb teeth that you are using. After the shower you can use a wide tooth comb to detangle you hair and then switch to a more fine tooth comb for styling. Or you can just try and finger comb first and see if there is actually any need for that transition.

Like I mentioned before, some men also have longer hair and may or may not use the tools that may seem like too much for us who cut our hair almost in a military fashion. But if you do need a straightening or a curling tool I think I'd suggest Enzo Milano. I must admit, I first liked it because it shared the name with one of the cars that I like, but after some research I found that they are also very good and innovative. Through the implementation of new design concepts and a commitment to delivering education on groundbreaking products, Renzo brought to life the extraordinary clipless curling iron that revolutionized professional appliances and provided a unique alternative to traditional flat and curling irons. No longer only for celebrities and Hollywood stylists, he is dedicated to injecting new life into the beauty product industry and has created a platform that has no barriers. There are, of course, not the only tools they offer.

I haven't tested this yet, but I believe I have a discount code for a few items, hope it still works. If you buy it through the shop use the code: enzo1319

Does hair product cause acne

I believe there isn't any product or anything for that matter that doesn't have some myth tied to it. Let's check the hair product causing acne. Can it do that?

Yes, it can, but it's not a rule. When we sleep, we sweat. Any product we have in our hair may then go on to our face. So that can cause the pores on the face to get clogged and eventually cause acne. Even worse if the product you are using is extra oily – ingredients like petroleum, jojoba oil, silicones and shea butter will be in those products. But solely this as a reason why you got acne is just too much. I would call this a semi-true statement. This is also one of the reasons why people block their forehead when applying hair spray. Gels, pomades and hairsprays tend to be the more irritating ones.

You could also be having an allergic reaction to an ingredient from the hair product that came in contact with your skin. So it's good to check what is in it every time. *Even though panthenol is actually a beneficial product some people report that using conditioners without it has decreased acne breakout.*

I would never suggest you don't use hair product at all. So the options are as follows: change your pillow very regularly, maybe even every day and if not every day, then maybe every day you use hair product; sleep only on your back; don't let the hair and the product touch your face and back of the neck or sleep with a *bonnet de douche.*

What ingredients you should avoid

I usually have some trust issues when people tell me that something is categorically good or bad, with nothing in between. Rarely something is as black or white, like that. We're not in a Green lantern movie… In brightest day, in blackest night, no evil shall escape my sight… This is why I suggest that when someone does give you such advice and they didn't really do the research, don't take that information for granted and as set in stone. It is their opinion. And guess what… It's just like those things on your body… everybody has one.

Sulfates will allegedly make your hair dry. These are the detergents that will strip your hair of its natural oils, but that is also the stuff that cleans it. This is why you will be using a conditioner too and you will get some nourishment back instantly. Detergents may also be interfering with all the ingredients beneficial for your hair, not allowing them to stay on it. There have been other studies regarding this ingredient. Actually, it is the harsher version of Sodium Lauryl Sulfate (SLS) that is linked with this. Even then, some say that it could cause mutations that could lead to forming of cancer. This is a lot of 'could's' and it is also provided that it is a stronger version and shampoos to my knowledge don't use those versions and the amount of sulfates isn't really that large. Some do claim that sulfates do not present any dangers as long as you do wash out your hair and do not leave any foam in it. What would be my advice on this? If possible, pass on the products that have SLS, but if not, do keep washing your hair. Sulfates can be helpful, they do remove grease and help you glide through the hair easier, but when buying a product look for a milder version of it, like *Sodium Lauryl Sulfoaccetate* and *Sodium Lauryl Sulfosuccinate*.

Parabens are a big one and you can see more and more products being made without them and they will advertise it too as paraben free. Parabens are used to prolong shelf life and in the ingredient list you will find them as methylparaben or propylparaben. They can irritate the skin and make the scalp unhealthy. There are also concerns that they are tied to cancer, developmental and reproductive ability. This is because they are found to mimic estrogen, which are found in breast cancer cells. In Denmark they are banned in the products for children up to 3 years old. They can reduce the sperm production and reduce testosterone levels. It is also an ingredient that will block the beneficial effects you may be going for, so you may very well be getting the negative effects without the positive ones. For 37 references just regarding parabens you can visit this website:

http://www.safecosmetics.org/get-the-facts/chemicals-of-concern/parabens/

Not all *alcohols* are bad (ask any alcoholic), some are actually beneficial for your hair. The good ones are the fatty alcohols that are derived from animals, plants or oils. They are used in products as emulsifiers, to mix oil and water. If you remember chemistry, oil and water don't usually mix together. They can actually add moisture instead of drying your hair out and do some other nice things too. So, which ones are good?

Good alcohols: Behenyl, Cetearyl, Cetyl, Lauryl, Myristyl, Stearyl.
Neutral alcohols: Benzyl (preservative), Propylene Glycol.
Bad alcohols: Ethanol, Isopropyl, Propanol, Propyl, SD Alcohol, SD Alcohol 40.

It's not just that these will damage your hair, Isopropyl is in anti freeze and it can cause headaches, dizziness, nausea, vomiting. No hair style is worth this.

Polyethylene Glycol or PEG is so harsh that this should be removing stains from a grill, not your hair. This is also a part of antifreeze.

Something else that deserves to stay in the kitchen is ***sodium chloride***. This is basically table salt. It is used in shampoos and conditioners that use SLS and they can dry out your scalp.

Silicone isn't all that bad as some of the other ingredients, but it does have a catch. If you have a product with silicones (dimethicone, cyclomethicone) you would need to use a shampoo with sulfates, which are powerful enough to strip it from your hair once in a while. If you do not remove them they could build up and while your hair appeared to be smoother will become greasier and weighed down.

Some websites mention ***chlorine*** as bad for your hair even though you can not find it in the products. Where you can find it is in your water. So unless you know how to influence what quality water you get for washing your hair it's beyond me what this means to anyone.

FD and C colour pigments is also something that was a subject of carcinogenic studies. Proven or not I tend to not use these products. If something claims that it has olive in it and has trouble being green without the colour, then I don't really want to even try it. Colour and *fragrance* should always be coming from the ingredients the product is using. If something is fragrance free this doesn't mean that it is also scent free, it only means that the fragrance is coming from the essential oils that were used for the production.

Proteins are another ingredient that aren't really bad for your hair, but you could overdo it with those. There is a saying that goes "Everything is a poison, it just depends on the dose". This is why I am suggesting to not use shampoos that have 1001 ingredients and forget about it. Proteins and some other things should come from within. You can not expect to have good hair just because you have a nice shampoo. There is what you eat, what you drink, how you sleep, do you work out, how high is your stress level, etc. If you overdose on protein your body may forget to produce it for your hair.

Another thing you should also avoid is *mineral oils*. But aren't oils good for you? Yes, oils usually are good for you, but let's check what mineral oils are. Mineral oil is a derivative of crude oil (petroleum) that is used industrially as a cutting fluid and lubricating oil. So, would you put some motor oil in your hair? Yeah, I guessed as much. Petrolatum exhibits many of the same potentially harmful properties as mineral oil. These will basically block your pores and prevent your skin to breathe, to take in nutrients and to get rid of toxins.

Dioxins are another ingredient I do not know how to present to you. It is found in antibacterial products and has some really bad side effects. It too is tied to cancer, changing of cells, etc. The problem is that this is not often or at all listed in the ingredients. If you want to see what dioxin poisoning does, just google "Ukrainian president dioxin poisoning".

DEA, MEA, TEA...What can I say, I wouldn't trust any ingredient that has the acronym of a Drug Enforcement Agency. DEAs (diethanolamine), MEAs (monoethanolamine) and TEAs (triethanolamine) are common ingredients in shampoos. They usually come with names like Cocamide MEA or DEA, or Lauramide DEA. Studies have shown that repeated skin applications of DEA based detergents can greatly increase your chance of liver or kidney cancer, and children are at an even greater risk. These are also known to disrupt chemicals in the body and form cancer-causing nitrates and nitrosamines. TEAs, one of the worst ingredients that is used to balance pH levels, cause allergic reactions including eye problems, dryness of hair and skin and can be toxic when absorbed into the body over time.

Formaldehyde, Quaternium-15 or Bronopol is basically the same thing. This is used to kill the bacteria and the FDA has approved it in small doses, but it is banned in Canada and some other countries. And let's face it, health Care in Canada is much better than the one in the States. Without me trying to list every bad thing that it does, just take the advice and stay clear from this ingredient.

As much as it may look like it in this article, I do not promote only natural products. I am aware that there are chemicals that are good and beneficial for our hair and skin. But you need to recognize which ones are which and make an educated choice on what you will be using as your product of choice. It will also be difficult to stay clear of all these ingredients, but at least now you know which to avoid and how to choose lesser of two evils.

Why does our hair gray – facts and myths

Generally, men have more gray hair than women. Asians and Africans have less gray hair than Caucasians. And for the Caucasians the Rule 50 applies – 50% Caucasians are 50% gray by the age of 50.

The most important thing to remember is that genes play a vital role in the greying of hair. In other words, if you have begun to notice grey hair, then it may be time you asked your parents when they first started spotting their grey hair.

But why does the hair turn gray? It doesn't. It grows gray. But kidding aside, that happens when the cells called melanocytes at the base of each hair follicle get damaged by exposure to the environment or something aggressive, disease or simply age. Exactly how hair loses its pigment remains unclear. In the early stages of graying, the melanocytes are still present but inactive. Later on they seem to decrease in number. Smoking can also accelerate the change of hair color, or lack thereof. The natural color of the hair depends on the distribution, type and the amount of melanin in he middle layer of the hair shaft or cortex. Hair has only two types of pigments: dark and light, and what color our hair gets is based on what kind of a mix of those two we get. Gray hair is simply hair with less melanin. There are other factors that can change the pigmentation of hair, making it lighter or darker. Scientists have divided them by internal and external factors; *internal factors*: genetic defects, hormones, body distribution, age; *external factors*: climate, pollutants, toxins, chemical exposure.

In general, *graying is not tied to any health conditions*. Early graying could be a sign of an autoimmune disease or heart disease, but please don't jump up right away to call a doctor, it is a symptom all of us have, but you can mention it on your next regular check. Stress is certainly a factor in going gray. Many parents will say they went gray because of their children. President Obama stated how much he aged and gained gray hair while he was in office. But while many do agree that stress is a factor, there is no measurable evidence to support it.

Hormones such as melanocyte-stimulating hormone can darken light hair, as can high levels of estrogen and progesterone, which are produced in pregnancy. Certain drugs such as those to prevent malaria can lighten hair, while some epilepsy medications can darken it.

Scientists have long known that in order to prevent hair from going grey they would need to either prolong the life of the melanocytes in the hair bulb – by protecting them from injury – or expand the melanocyte stem cell reservoir in the upper or top region of the hair follicle so they continue to replace lost pigment cells.

A group of French scientists have identified a new series of agents that protect hair follicle melanocytes from damage at the end of the hair cycle. This enables pigment production to restart as soon as the next hair cycle begins.

The agents work by mimicking the action of an enzyme called DOPAchrome tautomerase. This enzyme is the naturally occurring antioxidant in the hair bulb that protects melanocytes from oxidative damage. By duplicating the effects of DOPAchrome tautomerase, melanocyte metabolism and survival improves.

The new agents are being formulated into a product that can be applied as a spray-on serum or shampoo. But they won't re-colour grey hair or bring back the dead cells that produce hair colour. Instead, they protect your melanocytes.

The myths

There are more than two myths about the hair, but I didn't want to make the article too much longer, so I wanted to address two that need to be repeated.

If you pull out one gray hair, two more will grow in its place

Each hair on your head emerged from its own hair follicle. If a hair is plucked, the follicle can only hold one replacement.

A traumatic experience can cause your entire head of hair to go gray overnight

It is possible for a person's hair to appear to go gray overnight, but only if she has a rare condition such as alopecia areata, which may cause non-gray hair to fall out in large amounts before the gray hair does. This would make it seem like a person's hair turned gray overnight, when in reality it was hair loss that occurred—not color transformation.

Food good for your hair

Some nutritionists say that salmon is good for your hair if your hair is losing its natural shine. But honestly, with some of the fake colored salmon that is going around I would skip this one myself.

Pumpkin seeds are supposed to be good for a flaky scalp. These also benefit the prostate. So, men, I suggest you get these into your diet.

Rather than using products that contain ***protein***, you should eat something rich in protein. If you use a protein shampoo or a conditioner it can happen that the hair ODs on protein and the body forgets it needs to produce it. So you should eat ***chicken***.

For breaking hair it is good to eat something rich in ***vitamin C***. Vitamin C helps to create protein. *Vitamin C is good to consume with iron rich food.* Vitamin C helps iron absorb into the body. It is also an antioxidant. **NEVER** use the vitamin C from a drugstore. Only consume it from food like lemon, orange, strawberry, peppers. The drugstore vitamin C has 5-10 times more of the vitamin than the body can absorb and the part that doesn't get absorbed can be bad for you later on.

Apparently, if you are suffering from visible hair loss, ***beans*** are the way to go. These are rich in iron. When iron levels (serum ferritin) fall below a certain point, you may experience anemia. This disrupts the nutrient supply to the follicle, affecting the hair growth cycle and may result in shedding. Other food rich in iron is red meat, fish, lentil, spinach, broccoli, etc.

You will need vitamin A and E, minerals Zinc and Selenium. Before you go and buy this please go and consult your doctor or pharmacist, but in case you want to take some supplements for these, you could check out Centrum multivitamins. These actually have a decent amount of vitamin C, only 150% of the daily dose, compared to some 1000%. In combination with these you could ask for advice on something that doctors suggest for patients with liver failure. These can help your liver regenerate and work better in fighting toxins. Do not use this all the time. Especially if you do not drink alcohol or other medications. If you do, then occasionally this is even advised.

Consider using **oils**. Oil is not only good for your car and its health, it is also good for your health. Some are good to eat, some are good for a massage, some are good for both. So try if you can consume one tea spoon of some oil. If that sounds too bad, try and add it in a smoothie or some other natural drink. Some oils you could use are: olive oil, flax seed oil, coconut oil, pumpkin seed oil, etc.

A remedy that is used in some parts of the world is **Magnesium Chloride** ($MgCl_2$). It is one of those things that people attribute almost miracle-like effects. It is basically salt. Your table salt is Sodium Chloride (NaCl). Preparation is also simple. You boil 1 litre of water, let it cool down, pour it in a glass bottle and then dissolve the MgCl in that water. One small glass (shot glass) or even a bit less daily is enough. **Baking soda** can be used for quite a few things and is sometimes used for gastric acid problems, whitening or washing teeth etc. Baking soda is an alkaline so it is used to reduce the acidity of our organism. And since the acidity is also linked with our poor health and cancer, it's not bad to use every now and then. Don't overdo it, though.

Other food good for your hair:

- Eggs
- Nuts
- Avocados
- Beef
- Carrots
- Coriander
- Flax seeds

Teas good for your hair

If you have googled this then you have probably come across some advice where people are telling you to wash your hair with teas. Don't do that. Throughout these articles you will notice that I am saying that it isn't enough to work on your hair only from the outside. Find a nice shampoo and a conditioner and use those for washing your hair. Teas are made for drinking. Shoes are made for walking. And blogs are made for giving mad advice.

Sage is a traditional folk remedy for balding.
Nettles are rich in iron and essential minerals. It's good for circulation and it being a diuretic it stimulates urination and eliminates wastes that may be held in the body.
Rosemary also stimulates circulation.
Gingko biloba, native to China, also stimulates circulation. It helps relieve nervous tension and hair loss that is caused by stress.
Green tea is packed with antioxidants, it stimulates hair follicles and makes your hair grow faster. Panthenol is also present in green tea.
Lavender is known to fight all sorts of skin infections.
Oolong tea along with its other benefits promotes the growth of healthy hair.
Black tea is rich in caffeine and hair products that claim to fight hair loss are too. If caffeine is a problem for you then stick to the Oolong tea.

Apart from washing your hair with tea, what I also want you to avoid is drinking tea that is of a low quality. How will you know that a tea is a low quality product? Simple enough. If the filter bag has "tea dust" in it, then don't drink it. I'm not saying that this kind of tea will be bad for you, it probably won't. But it's not as good as if you were to find some tea that actually has leaves and flowers in those bags or even without bags.

So how do you use these teas? Well, same as with my cosmetics, I like to mix and match stuff and I do it with my teas also. I have my own mixtures for hair, skin and brain. You could make a mix of only a few if you find a shop that sells these teas. I sometimes go to 6 different teas in one mix.

Be sure to consult your… well, whatever the person selling tea is called… they will most likely know if some teas don't mix and match. These will mostly be based on the way they are prepared. Some teas may need to be in water for 2-3 minutes and some longer. Some maybe can't be boiled or are even made by infusing them over night in cold water.

And speaking of which… Never forget to drink enough water. Every cell in our organism demands water. We are made by large amount out of water. Water is a drink that can keep giving you energy and keep you energized even more than coffee if you switch those and drink only water for a while. Water is a very simple, yet very powerful drink.

Apart from its healing qualities as a healing herb, enjoying a cup of tea can also be a very calming experience, your daily ritual even bordering on meditation. I am not suggesting you pick up *chado* or anything, but if you allow yourself a moment in the day for this small ceremony you will effectively be fighting the fast lifestyle we are used to living and you will be fighting stress. Unlearn that the stress and fast lifestyle are normal.

Stress

I am sick and tired of people telling you that everything is because you are under stress. Ironically, putting me under stress. It's not that I don't believe that stress can do that, it's just that sometimes people use it as a go to answer when they cannot explain what is wrong with you.

Sometimes people will tell you that hair falling out because of stress is a myth. Which is not correct. I have seen stress affect people in many negative ways and influence their health and hair is no different. Stress leads to a temporary hair loss condition called telogen effluvium. This condition causes the hair to fall out and when the hair grows back, it's often less pigmented than the original, and can eventually turn gray. In 2011, a study by Nobel Prize winner Robert Lefkowitz discovered that long-term productions of the body's fight or flight response—the instinctive ability to mobilize energy in response to a threatening situation—can damage your DNA and cause premature aging, including graying hair.

Mental and physical stress can certainly have an impact on your hair falling out and regrowth. Persistent illness, drastic weight loss, physical labor... Basically anything that can cause your body to dehydrate can make the hair follicles undernourished and weak and cause hair loss.

But how do you fight something as invisible as stress? Try to introduce some calmness into your life. Do you have people who make you angry when you are around them? Do not call them anymore or do not answer the phone when they do. Do you have a political show you like to watch, but end up yelling at the TV? Try not to watch it. For your overall health, not just your hair, it can be beneficial if you are a borderline phlegmatic. If nothing is really touching you that much.

Other than avoiding stressful situations and stressful people what can you do? Well, you can always try to meditate. Meditation is a very good tool and exercise for the brain and the spirit. You focus on your breathing and imagine the world a bit better place and what you want to achieve. Maybe it's a result at work or school, maybe it's just hair growth, doesn't matter. Before meditation you could have a cup of chamomile tee, since it does have a calming effect.

Some people think they are too manly for meditation. Well, I believe they will change their minds in time, but until they do and they need something more physical to calm down, then I suggest the martial art Aikido. It is a defensive martial art that, if you find a right school, also focuses on breathing and controlling, leading, instead of forcing. I suggest the Aikikai school style, which should be a healthy combination of everything you need.

Exercise

Exercise will benefit your health in more ways than one. It will benefit your cardiovascular system, it will be good for your muscle tonus, your shape and having your muscles finally appear can also be beneficial for your self-image and confidence, sleeping better, increasing your happiness, which in turn also can benefit your health by fighting stress. All of these directly or indirectly have benefits to your hair.

Let's see how else exercise can help your hair:

- *It will get rid of toxins.* You will remove those toxins through sweating, especially while doing cardio exercises. This will make your sebum purer and more able to healthily condition your hair.
- *It will improve your posture.* Funnily enough, this can also affect the health of your scalp and your hair because a good posture also means a good blood flow and circulation to your scalp.
- *Exercise can help balance out hormones*, especially sex hormones such as testosterone or the human growth hormone (HGH). Hormonal problems, in turn, are linked to issues such as poor skin and poor hair growth. Take care of one, you take care of the other. This is especially true in males, where regular exercise has been shown to improve testosterone levels by 25 percent and nearly quadruple HGH levels. Well-balanced hormones can prevent thinning or unhealthy hair growth, and exercise is one of the best way to balance out those hormones.

Switch your exercise around, don't always do the same thing. So, while moderate to high cardio is suggested, I would also say that it would reap more benefits if you switch them sometimes. If you're combining cardio and calisthenics usually, then add swimming once a week. But other than exercise, you should also treat yourself with a sauna, halo therapy (relaxing in a salt room), massage every now and then. Think of a period how often you should do that and it should probably be shorter than that. My suggestion? At least one massage a month, one sauna a month, one salt room therapy every three months.

While exercise is great, you should take into consideration that there can also be too much of the good thing. This can be too much for two reasons: *stress* and *sweat*. People who exercise too much could be too focused on their looks and stressed that they aren't loosing weight or looking a certain way and this in turn affects the general health and the quality of the hair. Too much exercise also causes you to sweat too much, sweat contains salt and salt build up on your scalp can cause it to dry out.

SKIN

Daily skin routine for men

I have mentioned this already in some detail at the start of this brochure, so I may be repeating myself a little here, so please bear with me here.

As men we aren't really used to using skin care products and our daily skin routine for far too long consisted only out washing our faces with any soap we could find. Anyone who was using something more was labelled *metrosexual*… at least. Today this term has almost died out because of how much we actually accepted this as normal, so there is no more need for it. And why shouldn't we? It's a good and healthy habit.

But what should that habit entail for us men? Probably more products than you would like, but skin being our largest organ, we should take better care of it, while we can. Once the damage happens, it is much worse trying to heal it or mask it, instead of avoiding it all together. So, let's see what would be this somewhat over the top, but needed routine:

Every man should use a face wash instead of regular soap. Even if you aren't using the bar soap that has touched who knows what part of your body, the liquid soap could be too cheap and too aggressive for you to use on your skin and rely on it to take good care of it.

Every now and then *you should be using a face scrub*. This will help you remove dead cells from your face. This is something you wouldn't be using every day, try three times a week, would probably be best to have certain days when you are using this, to be able to better keep the routine.

After the face wash you should use a *day cream*. A day cream usually has some sort of SPF (sun protection factor) and some other nourishing ingredients. If you don't dry your face completely after washing it, you should need less of the day cream and it should spread easier across your face. Also, these creams usually have ingredients that keep moisture in your skin, so it wouldn't be bad to have some of the moisture on it when applying it.

Depending on your age and how you treated your skin, you may want to add an *eye cream* to your routine just for the crows feet that you may or may not have.

The next face wash should be in the evening. If you used the scrub today, you don't use it again. You also don't use your day cream, no need for SPF when there is no sun out. So, the only difference here is that *instead of the day cream, you will be using the one for the night time.* You can use the eye cream again now.

Do not wash your face too often. Even if you have an oily face, try and control yourself. If you wash your face 15 times a day, you are removing its natural oils and it in turn is producing it to combat the dryness. Doing this you are basically training your face to produce the excess of oil you are so trying to avoid. So, wash your face only twice daily. There are two options here for you – either wash your face in the morning and in the evening; or wash your face when you go out and when you get back into the house (obviously, don't mean after 5 minutes in your back yard). The reason that I am saying this is because wherever you are, the air has at least some pollution, dust, exhaust fumes, sweat, product you put on when you got out… all this is mixing and staying on your skin, possibly clogging your pores. Rather than waiting for the evening to wash your face, you can do it as soon as you get back. And it's even not that bad to give the face a little break until you apply the night cream. Instead of washing your face with product before applying the cream, you could just splash some water on your face and then apply the cream.

Remember that your lips are on your face too, so you need to take care of those too if you don't want to lick your lips every 3 seconds like LL Cool J. Menscience is on a pricier side, but offers SPF of 30, but Anthony may be somewhat more appealing since it's more affordable. You probably won't like this idea, but you could also try using a face mask once in a while. You determine how often you are comfortable using one – once a week, month, whatever. They even make some that are supposedly for men and the sheet form of the mask makes it incredibly easy to use. You could use a manual or electrical face wash brush and there is even another tool that could help you clear your face and get more tonus in it, it's called a PMD.

Food good for your skin

What we eat can affect our skin in more ways than just one. First of all, eating healthily will increase our overall health and our body and its functions will be working better, hence clearing the organism of various toxins, etc. Apart of having a healthy body, food can also affect our hormone levels and cause acne and other skin changes. This is why we should be eating foods that will boost our immunity, give us energy, clean our organism and feed our skin.

Sometimes people will tell you to stop eating chocolate. Well, that isn't really true. Or not 100% at least. Dark chocolate with higher levels of cocoa is actually good for you, not only your skin. Cocoa hydrates your skin, making it firmer and more supple and it also contains flavonols, which are a potent antioxidant. It is up to you, but it would probably be best to eat one row a day of 70% and higher cocoa content chocolate.

Me giving you permission to eat a certain kind of chocolate is not something you should adopt universally. Please be advised that too much sugar in your food, just like too much of anything, can be bad. So, if you can satisfy your need for sugar with dark chocolate, that's great. If you can't, please try some replacements for it. Sugar can have a withdrawal period, but once you get clean, you will not be able to recognize yourself.

You could add protein to you diet by eating a yogurt every now and then. The Greek yogurt is supposed to be richer in protein and if mixed with honey is a real health benefit. Red, orange and darker fruits and vegetables are usually great for skin, containing, among other things, carotene.

Tomatoes are rich in lycopene, a potent antioxidant that protects skin from UV damage.

You could also consider using some of the food supplements. One of those is chlorella. Chlorella is a green algae that has certain good benefits to your health and skin, but comes at a price... the taste or smell isn't the best, so instead of drinking them in form of a pill, you could buy the powder version and mask it in some good smoothie. Be sure to get the one that has a broken cell wall.

Some oils are also great to use. Two very good ones are coconut oil and olive oil. Olive oil was used on skin for many years and those cultures certainly knew what they were doing. So, while olive oil is great on the skin too, you can also eat it, but it isn't advised to use it on high temperatures. Maybe best to use it in salads or even just take a small spoon by itself. On the other hand, coconut oil is also great to eat and it doesn't discriminate any heat levels, but don't use it too much on your body if you have problems with acne.

Very often I see people suggest salmon as good for your skin and health in general. I'm a little bit skeptical because of the issues with farmed salmon and people even colouring the salmon or what not. So, while I do agree that you need to get omega-3 acids, you could ask around and see what other fish is good that you can get in your area or you could always get it as a supplement in form of a capsule.

Avocado is full of healthy fats that benefit our body in general, including the skin. I am not the biggest fan of raw avocado, but I'll take a few pieces while preparing it for a smoothie. I would add an avocado, a banana, walnuts, pumpkin seeds, coconut oil, 1 tea spoon or the hotel packaging of honey, 1 clove of garlic and maybe some super food you may have handy like goji berries or something else.

Add the rest according to how you like your smoothies – with water, ice or yogurt. To be honest, my drinks rarely taste good, but they are a health bomb.

Other food that is good for your skin:
- Pomegranate
- Walnuts
- Peppers
- Almonds
- Broccoli
- Kidney beans
- Eggs

Teas good for your skin

Coffee can also be good for your skin, but it is important not to overdo it with anything. Recently I have seen a Dr. Oz show where someone argued how good 2, 4, 6, etc. cups of coffee are. Well, first of all, not all coffee is created equal and some has a greatly reduced quality, while others may be great. You get what you pay. And the other thing is… When do the downsides start to outweigh the upsides? So, OK, it's possible that several cups of coffee can reduce risk of a certain disease or cancer, but when do these people who drink 6 and more cups of coffee a day sleep?!

It is not much different with teas. I would advise to drink tea twice a day at most, not more. No matter how much fluids you get in during the day through coffee, tea, juice, etc., it is also important to have a source of pure water and drink several glasses a day. Skin doesn't only need to be hydrated from the outside, but from the inside as well. If you can avoid the tea dust, buy tea leaves. If the filter dust is all you can get, that's better than nothing, but if possible, go for higher quality.

In the world of teas, green tea may be one of the wider known and most appreciated teas from the "general public", but while green tea is great, there are more potent teas that affect our skin, such as white tea. I am not advocating against green tea, if anything, I would advocate to mix the teas, so you don't need to drink 10 cups, like I would end up doing if I wasn't mixing my teas.

If you want to use chamomile, I would avoid drinking it. Maybe use its vapor to open and clear your pores as the tea is actually calming. Because its calming effects some studies have shown that people who drank chamomile had slower brain functions. I wouldn't say it alters them, it's just the calming sleepy effect of chamomile.

These are the teas that I would suggest. If you have a shop that holds these, it would be best to speak to someone working there and tell you how you can best mix these teas. Or, if you prefer, take just one, I just love mixing them.

- Green tea
- White tea
- Black tea
- Rooibos
- Jasmine
- Dandelion
- Oolong
- Burdock

How to shave

Again, we spoke about shaving at the beginning, so I hope you will stay with me here while we try to go through it in a little bit more detail and somewhat bigger font.

What do we need to know about shaving? Well, we could start with the tools we would be using and how to choose those. Today there are so many razors with flexible heads, multiple blades, etc. My advice is to avoid those. If you must use, I guess I'd suggest Harry's, but… I hope you go with something that has less blades. And I would suggest either a double edge safety razor or if you are a bit more bold – a shavette. A shavette is a straight razor that doesn't have a blade you need to sharpen, but instead uses the same blades as the safety razor.

I use a safety razor. Even though shaving should be a process and a ritual I like that it goes safer and faster with it. Plus, I only shave with my right hand, so I don't like how I obscure my view and what shapes and angles I have to do with my hand when shaving with a shavette. Also, I found that I press down harder when the razor head moves too much, so I prefer minimum movement or none.

Apart from that, you will need a little bit more still. You could have some kind of a trimmer or something that you could use to shorten your beard to have an easier time shaving it. You would need a brush to apply the shaving cream to your face. Using your palm it can happen that you flatten your beard and the brush specifically avoids that. In some states in the USA you will find that those are forbidden in barber shops because it's impossible to sterilize those. You could buy yourself some kind of a soap dish, but it's not really that needed. When I'm a bit lazy to clean too much afterwards or when I'm in a hurry, I'll foam the cream up in my palm even.

What would you need from the products? You need a face wash. It would be great if it had some kind of antibacterial in it because you are preparing for shaving and cuts may happen. It's not bad to exfoliate once in a while also, so you could get that, but I wouldn't call it a must-have for shaving. As a pre-shave product I prefer a pre-shave cream instead of pre-shave oil. After the pre-shave product apply the shaving cream and then shave.

I prefer the cream because it doesn't have some ingredients you really shouldn't be putting on your skin, that gels and foams use as a propellant. And the difference with soap is that you can get it easier on the brush and foam faster, while soap is harder and you may need a dish for it.

I personally do three passes. First time I shave top to bottom and never pass the same spot twice once I removed the cream from that spot. Wash my face with water only. Apply cream and do a second pass. Now the shaving goes as much as possible from side to side. Or from the ears towards the nose. Same direction on the neck. Wash the face again and apply cream again. Now shave bottom to top. Wash face, inspect if you missed something and fix if needed. If you did cut yourself somewhere, don't use the toilet paper, buy yourself a styptic that is used to stop the bleeding.

Since I do have somewhat sensitive skin, I don't like using after shaves with too much alcohol in them, so I use balms or some other cream that I use for my face. I don't use or suggest anyone used a hand cream, which I've seen people do.

VARIOUS THOUGHTS

What should you know about perfume

First thing you should know… Not everything is a perfume. That's why most of the time we are talking about scents or fragrances. First I will tell you a bit about the classification. More than you will want to know, but still… There are many men out there who think cologne is for men and perfume for women. So let's see… *Eau Fraiche* has 1-3% of perfume oil in alcohol and water. It lasts under an hour. *Cologne or Eau de Cologne* has 2-4% perfume oils in alcohol and water. Usually last for two hours. *Eau de Toilette* has 5-15% pure perfume essence dissolved in alcohol. Usually lasts for three hours. *Eau de Parfum* has 15-20% pure perfume essence and can last 5 to 8 hours. *Perfume*, not edp, has 20-30% pure perfume essence and can last to 24 hours.

Less is more. Sometimes too much of the good thing can be as offensive as actually smelling really bad. And there is no rule that is set in stone. Apply to pulse points on your neck and wrists – with pulse points, the blood flow is more and the heat dissipates the scent and spreads it. Me personally, I give it four squirts – wrists and sides of neck. But you'll need to test this and make a decision based on how strong the fragrance is. Learn how the cologne reacts to your chemistry and body.

Do **NOT** pat or rub the perfume, heat you create makes it evaporate faster. Do not apply to the clothes. Do not apply to your hair, even though it can hold the scent longer because it's greasy. Do not use any creams after the perfume, those you will need to use before. Do not use just any perfume, learn what season it is for and is it a night or day perfume. DO NOT use the cloud method to apply perfume. You're just wasting the perfume to create a cloud to walk through hoping that something will stick to you.

There are some questions to be asked when you get to the shop. If you like to follow trends, that question would be *'what's new'*. You may want to see *what is popular*. Now, you can make this a question that will be in favor of buying or against. Why against? Because if it's popular many people may be buying it. You could ask... but watch out if the boyfriend or husband is around... *what is your favorite*? You're buying it for yourself and you want to like it and you want everyone else to like it too, but most of all you want the ladies to like it.

Should you spray the perfume on you? I wouldn't. I always get a few of those paper thingies and test it there. The fragrance reacts a little bit different with paper than it would with your skin, but if you have a pen you can write a few letters on the paper and check it later on too. And you will probably be wearing something anyway, so you don't want to mix those.

What is the optimal number of perfumes you should try? You don't want to sniff perfumes until you get dizzy. So *5 would be the most you would try*, but I would keep it at up to 3. The reason is that you do not want to lose track what you tried and have the scent from the first 15 now interfere with the scent you're trying to test on number 16. Do not oversaturate your nose and your brain with too many fragrances. Some shops will even have coffee beans for you to smell before you go on to the next one, but still keep the number low.

After all the testing, you should get out. Give it some time to set and see how it fades. Have a cup of coffee or something. After that, go back to the store and if you still like it, buy that one. Why should you not buy it right away? Fragrances have 3 types of notes. A top note, a medium note and a base note. When one of the notes evaporates the one "underneath" it comes to show. So you want to experience the fragrance before you decide on it.

How to find the perfume that you love? You could always give a try to Scentbird if you are from the USA. On their website you'll find all kinds of different fragrances. Some of them I actively avoid, some are not something I would consider brands that should be making those, but some I think are great and if you don't know what fragrance to commit to, this is a great way to test it. Sometimes a short visit to a shop isn't enough to decide if you like something or not, so having a smaller bottle to *date a perfume before marrying it*, as they say on their website, is helpful. Great thing about them is that, unlike some subscription sales, they also offer a one time purchase.

The ones I don't like are fragrances like Mercedes. Great cars, think they should stick to those. I also wasn't a fan of Dolce and Gabana The One, but I didn't try the light blue version. But what I do like on their website and what I would love to try out are the following fragrances:
- MALIN+GOETZ Cannabis (didn't try, would love to see what it is like)
- Bvlgari Aqva
- Bvlgari Aqva Amara
- Hugo Boss Just different

These are some of the other fragrances I liked:
- Bvlgari BLV
- Bvlgari Black
- Bvlgari Aqva, the first original one
- Davidoff Cool Water
- Paco Rabane Invictus
- Calvin Klein Euphoria
- Armani Code

- Armani Attitude
- I did not have the pleasure of using Cartier L'Envol for a longer period of time, but it seemed nice, I did like it

Not sure if you noticed, but I do seem to like Bvlgari a lot. It took a lot for me not just to list all of the Bvlgari products. Should probably ask for a perfume or something. Actually, would rather prefer the ring Zero.

You may love a certain kind of perfume and I have been in the same situation more than once, but you really should change it sometimes. Even if you buy two at once, one that you like and one that you're getting for a change. Change is good, you want to keep it fresh. Maybe your girlfriend recognizes the perfume you were wearing on your first date or something. It happened to me, why wouldn't it happen to you. So you can buy a smaller bottle of that perfume and still have it, but just switch it up a bit sometimes.

What do the symbols on the containers represent

Sometimes the packaging of the cosmetics has some kind of symbols that we have no idea what they are representing. There's so many of those and some just mean the same thing.

Period After Opening (PAO)

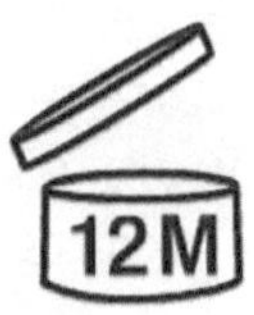

Products that have a shelf life longer than 30 months are required to have this icon. This icon is represented by an open jar, which usually has a number on it. Sometimes the number is in a different place. The number is representing the number of months that the period should be good for after you open it. This shouldn't be confused that the product will go bad after that period, but it can happen that some of its chemical properties start to change and it can't guarantee the scent or effect as it would be prior to that date.

Best Before End Of

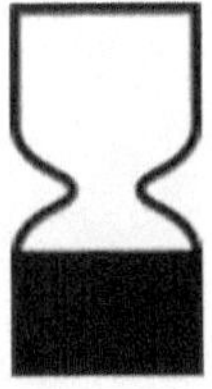

Products that have a shelf life shorter than 30 months need to have a best before date on the label. It can be symbolized by an hourglass or an egg timer and is abbreviated BBE or Exp. Like the previous one, it is only required in the EU for now.

Further information

It is not common for a cosmetic product to have something that you need to read before you start using it, but some do. Those are most likely rated as cosmeceutical. That is represented by this symbol. Most everything that has additional information provided with it is smart to read in case it can cause allergies or dryness of the skin, irritation, can't mix with some of the medications that you are using or if you have a cold, some other health condition, are pregnant, etc.

Estimated

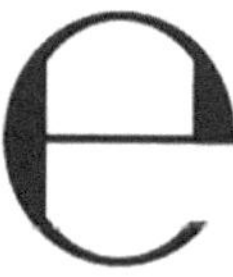

Estimated is probably one of the most dishonest symbols is any industry. This symbol mostly appears after the amount of product is written on the packaging. So, if they say that a product has 100 ml, they don't actually say it has 100 ml, they say they estimate it has that amount, but it could have more or, more likely, less than that.

Green dot

Green dot, which isn't always green, is representing that the manufacturer pays to recover and recycle the product.

Flammable

This is pretty much self-explanatory. Products with this picture on them are not to be stored near any heat sources, used near an open flame or expose in any way to high heat. These are mostly the pressurized kind of products like hair sprays, deodorants, etc.

Some rabbits

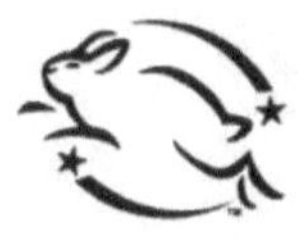

There are also symbols that are pretty much used for the same thing. The rabbit symbol says that the product isn't tested on animals and is

therefore cruelty free. And that would be the regular leaping rabbit. For some reason, unknown to me, there is a symbol for the same thing, but by PETA now. The same symbol is used with addition of text to say that the product is not only cruelty free, but also vegan.

Mobius loop

Mobius loop is a symbol that can tell us three things. One, we don't know what a Mobius loop is. Two, if the symbol is inside a circle, then it means that it is made from recycled material. In case there is a % number inside the symbol or near it, then that means that the packaging is made from that amount of recycled material. Three, if it's just a Mobius loop without any additional symbols, then that means that the container is recyclable.

The Tidy Man

Even though some may have confused him in the past as a symbol for recycling or something related to that, this symbol is actually a warning to us to be more responsible and dispose of the waste responsibly.

Organic cosmetics

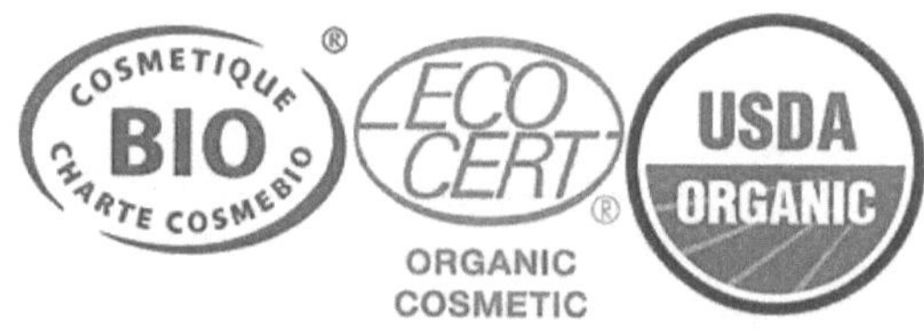

The French organization, COSMEBIO, has a couple symbols for cosmetic labels depending on the product's certification. The BIO symbol stands for "biologique" (organic) and signifies that the product contains at least 95% natural ingredients, and that organic farming account for at least 10% of the total products and 95% of the plant ingredients. The ECO symbol symbol stands for "ecologique" (natural) and tells consumers that the product contains at least 95% natural ingredients, and that organic farming accounted for at least 5% of the total product and 50% of the plant ingredients.

The Ecocert Organic symbol is from a nongovernmental certification program that evaluates the organic contents of products. Labels with the Ecocert Organic symbol signify that the product has at least 95% plant-based ingredients, and at least 10% of all its ingredients by weight are organic. If the product has an Ecocert Natural symbol, that means at least 50% of the ingredients are plant-based, and at least 5% of all its ingredients by weight are organic.

The seal indicates that at least 95% of the product's ingredients are organic. Manufacturers have to be certified by the United States Department of Agriculture (USDA) to be legally able to use the seal on product labels and packaging.

Resin

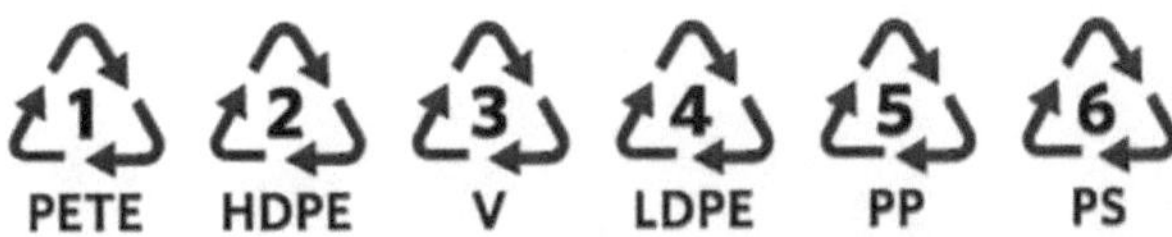

Usually seen on plastics, the SPI (Society of the Plastics Industry) resin identification coding system is used to identify polymer types when recycling. This is very important when labeling packaging because just one wrong item could potentially ruin a batch during the recycling process. Plastics are recycled according to the resin type, and the recyclables are either hand sorted, or done through a process of shredding and separating through air or liquid density separation. Plastics must be sorted according to this system in order for the final product to be usable.

polyethylene terephthalate	high-density polyethylene	polyvinyl chloride	low-density polyethylene	polypropylene	polystyrene
soft drink bottles, mineral water, fruite juice container, cooking oil	milk jugs, cleaning agents, laundry detergents, bleaching agents, shampoo bottles, washing and shower soaps	trays for sweets, fruit, plastic packing (bubble foil) and food foils to wrap the foodstuff	crushed bottles, shopping bags, highly-resistant sacks and most of the wrappings	furniture, consumers, luggage, toys as well as bumpers, lining and external borders of the cars	toys, hard packing, refrigerator trays, cosmetic bags, costume jewellery, CD cases, vending cups

Should men use female products

No.

Other publications by Davor Pavlic

The cosmetics entrepreneur manual: The first complete book about starting a cosmetics business
https://www.amazon.com/dp/1973447614

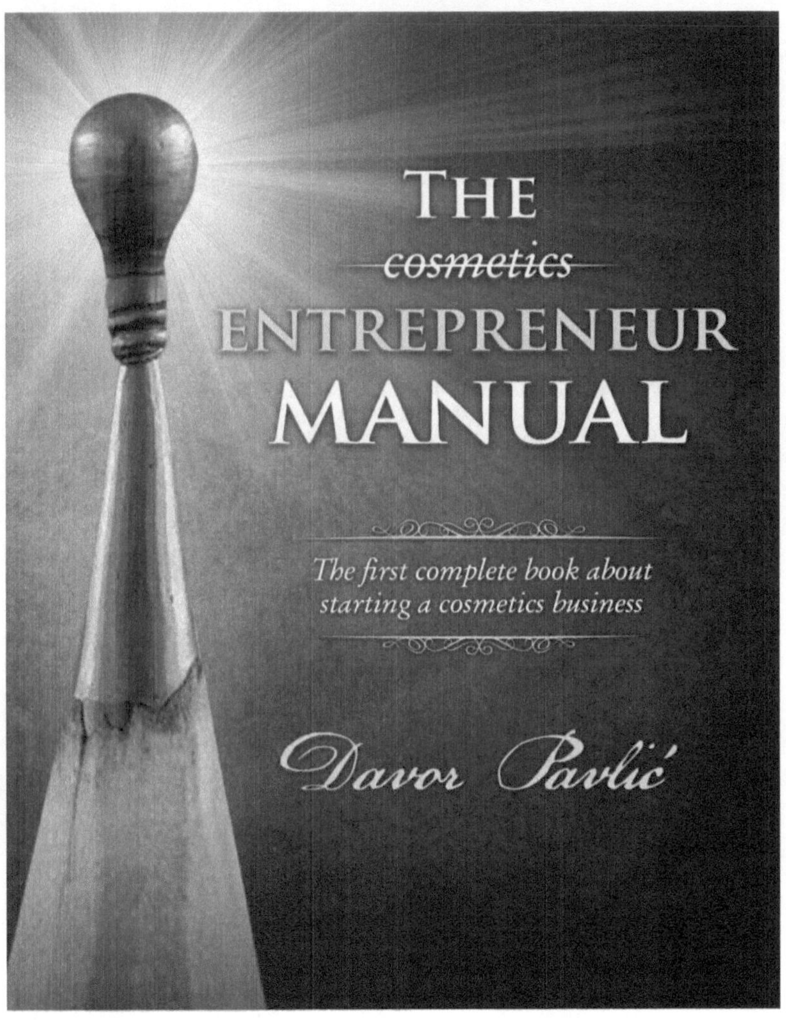